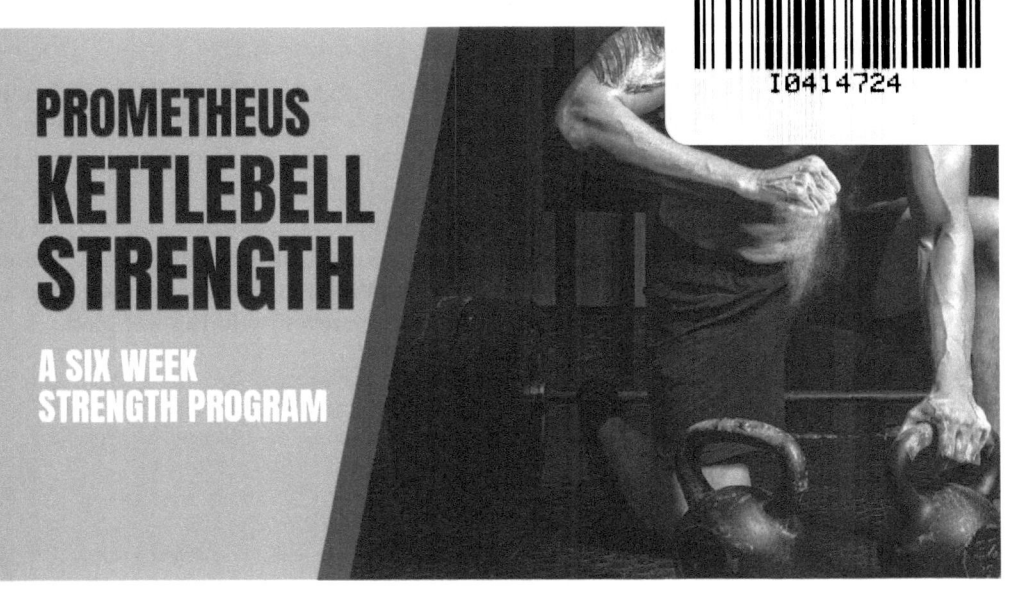

Prometheus

Kettlebell Strength Program

A six-week kettlebell strength program that can be completed with a single kettlebell. The program is simple and based on three super-powerful kettlebell exercises that work the full-body.

Everything you need to complete the workout and program is covered in this book, warm-ups, exercise descriptions, photos, how to adjust the program, alternative exercises, muscle priming, and even a bonus video of the workout so you can see how to execute the movements.

In Greek mythology, Prometheus is a Titan, who is credited with the creation of man from clay, and who defies the gods by stealing fire and giving it to humanity, an act that enabled progress and civilization. In our kettlebell world, Prometheus is going to be your progression in strength.

About the author

My name is Taco Fleur, and I'm a Russian Girevoy Sport Institute Kettlebell Coach, IKFF Certified Kettlebell Trainer, Kettlebell Level 1 + 2 Trainer, Kettlebell Science and Application, CrossFit Level 1 Trainer, CrossFit Judges Certificate, CrossFit Programming Certificate, MMA Conditioning Level 1, MMA Fitness Level 1 + 2, Punchfit Trainer and Plyometrics Trainer Certified, with a purple belt in Brazilian Jiu Jitsu. Author on BoxRox and featured in 4 issues of the Iron Man magazine. I have owned and set-up 3 functional kettlebell gyms in Australia and Vietnam, and lived in the Netherlands, Australia, Vietnam and Thailand. I'm currently living in Spain.

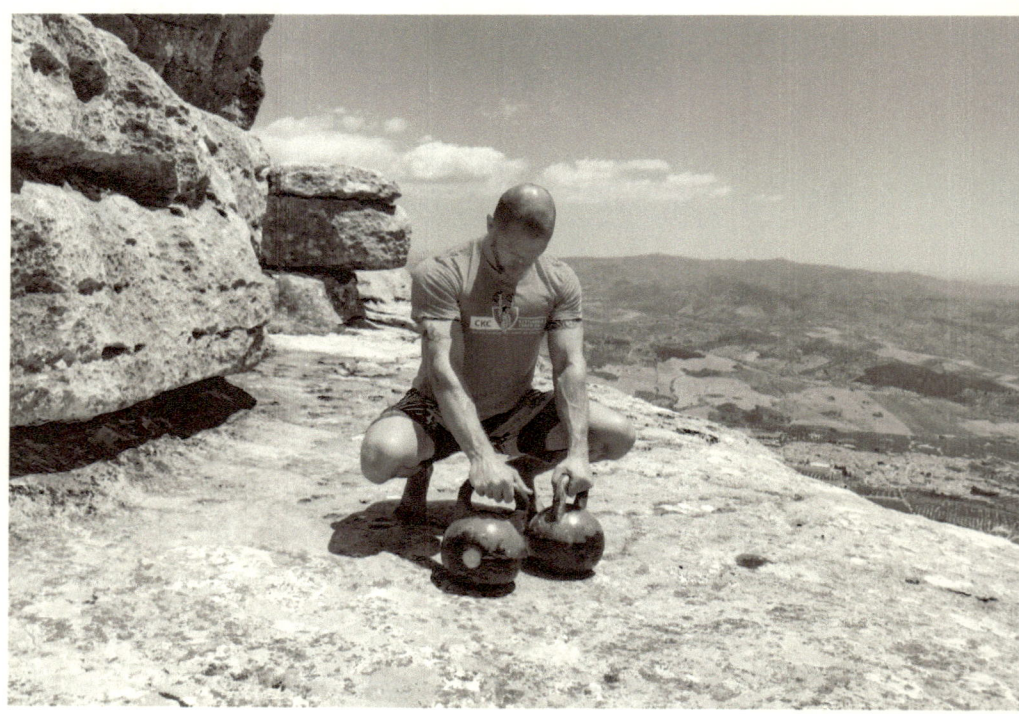

The first thing I'd like you to know about me is that I do **not** know everything, I don't pretend to know everything, and I never will. I'm on a path of life-long learning. I believe there is always something to learn from someone, no matter who they are. I've been physically active since the day I arrived on this earth in 1973. I got serious about training in 1999, touched a kettlebell for the first time in 2004, and got serious about kettlebell training in 2009. I'm here to do what I love most, and that is to share my knowledge with the world.

Some of my personal bests are 1 hour unbroken clean and jerk with a 16kg; 40 minutes unbroken clean and jerk with a 20kg; 400 burpees performed within one hour; 500 kettlebell snatches, 500 swings, and 500 double-unders completed in one session; 250 alternating dead clean and presses in one session with 20kg; 200 pull-ups in one session; 200 unbroken kettlebell swings with a 28kg; most kettlebell swings completed in one session with a 28kg (1,501); most total kettlebell swings done in 28 days with a 28kg (11,111); windmill with a 40kg kettlebell; lugged a kettlebell up a 3,479m mountain; 160kg dead lift; 100 snatches on sand with a 24kg kettlebell; 85kg Olympic Squat Snatch; 300 unbroken clean and jerk with 20kg kettlebell; 10 minute unbroken clean and jerk 80 reps with 2 x 16kg kettlebells; 532 unbroken snatches and achieved rank 2 in kettlebell sport. I mention these PBs not to boast but to demonstrate that I have a good understanding of technique and movement across different areas.

My own training and goals are geared around GPP (General Physical Preparedness) which involves kettlebell training, calisthenics and CrossFit. I like high-volume reps but also like greasing the groove now and again. My main goals are to remains as agile as possible, remaining mobile, training in as many planes of movements as possible, and learning as many different exercise combinations and movements as possible while having fun and enjoying Brazilian Jiu Jitsu. I'm no Arnold Schwarzenegger and never will be, but strength is not solely defined by physical appearance and huge bulging muscles.

You can read more about my training, philosophy, and other ramblings on my website, www.cavemantraining.com, and on my YouTube channel, bit.ly/youtube-cavemantraining, which as of this writing has over 36,000 subscribers and more than 5 million views.

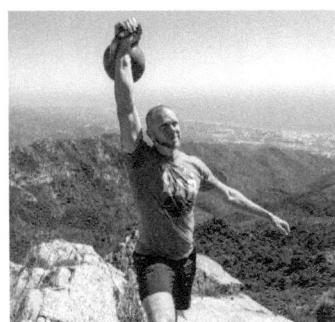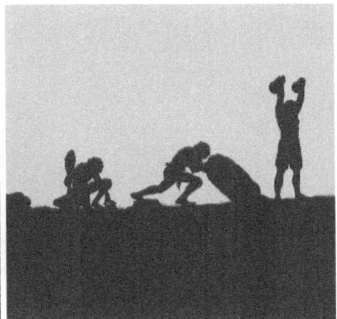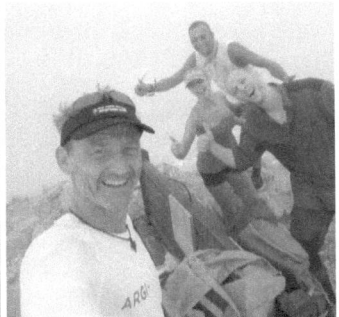

Add me: Facebook.com/taco.fleur or Facebook.com/coach.taco.fleur
Instagram: *@realcavemantraining*

Facebook.com/Cavemantraining or Facebook.com/Cavemantraining.Magazine
for up-to-date articles and news.

Note: Most of the kettlebell stock images used in this book have literally been created with blood, sweat, and tears - I'm talking about lugging kettlebells for hours up mountains, through canyons, running out of water to drink, etc. Please respect the effort that has gone into producing the photos.

Photos are available for purchase, or in some cases made available for educational purposes with appropriate credits/links in return.

CAVEMANTRAINING

Table of Contents

Results

Some of the results you can expect when completing this program correctly are, but not limited to:

- Increase of overall strength
- Shoulder strength
- Leg strength
- Core strength
- Hip strength
- Arm strength
- Calf strength
- Increase of overall flexibility
- Shoulder stability
- Overall hypertrophy
- Triceps hypertrophy
- Quadriceps hypertrophy
- Latissimus hypertrophy
- Deltoids hypertrophy
- Increase of self-confidence

The most important factors that will allow you to obtain these results are consistency, persistence, safety, nutrition, rest, mindset, form and technique, good connection and activation of the required muscles, and most of all leaving the ego at the door.

Number of kettlebells required

You could complete the program with just one kettlebell, you could even complete it with a lighter than recommended kettlebell. There is always going to be a positive result at the end of the program no matter what. The optimal number of kettlebells is two, both heavy, but one being heavier. Most people will be able to row and swing more than they can get overhead. In the bonus video, I demonstrate the workout with the BEAST (48kg/106lb) for the swings and rows and use a 32kg/70lb for the jerks.

What weight to start with

The weight to start with should be around 60 to 80% of your 1 rep max. I'd like to say 80% but it will really depend on your conditioning and technique. So, you can also look at this and grab the heaviest weight that allows you to complete the full workout without sacrificing form or technique. If you grab a weight that will affect your form on round 2 or 3 then you've picked one that's too heavy or you've not rested enough. With that said, no amount of rest within a normal session is going to work if you picked a weight too heavy.

Alternative exercises

Some alternative exercises or regressions are, push press instead of a jerk, and dead swing instead of swings. The push press is the progression to the jerk, hence, a great option to regress to. The dead swing means you bring the kettlebell dead to the ground upon each rep. You'll want to use this alternative if you're stuck with a weight that might be a little bit too heavy. The return to dead upon each rep gives your lower back a break and allows you to rest and reset between reps.

Why the rep range

The rep range is kept low with rest to allow you to put everything in each rep, to never sacrifice form, and to be able to work more often rather than walking away with aches and pains that you need to recover from, meaning you're out of action, you're not training. You could do 3 sessions and double the reps of which the risk of putting you over that edge is higher, or you do 5 sessions with lower reps and keeping you safer, I choose the latter. Over time you will you also get more volume in by increasing sessions.

Adjust the program

If you have a lighter kettlebell than is recommended there are ways to make the program work for you as best as possible. You can switch from double arm to single-arm swings and double the reps, i.e. 4 reps done with double arm will turn into 4 reps on one arm and 4 on the other arm. If you have two kettlebells that are lighter than one of the recommended weights then you can use double kettlebell swing. This does require you to take a wider stance but you're still hitting the recommended load. If your weight is currently too heavy for you then you can change the swing to a dead swing which means the kettlebell comes back to dead upon each rep. This is great to put a little pause in between reps and reset. It's also great if you want to work on power.

The jerk is an advanced exercise and can be replaced with the push press. A push press is where you use your legs to get the weight up with only one knee jerk and follow through with a press out. A push press or jerk allows you to get heavier weight overhead and more often than you would with a strict press.

Warm-up

Always warm-up prior to your workout. The areas to focus on in particular are the calves, hamstrings, quadriceps, hip flexors, erector spinae, deltoids, and everything else around the shoulder area.

10 x jumping jacks

6 x squats

4 x hip hinges

The above is a basic warm-up you can use for 4 to 8 minutes. If you're also going to use the muscle priming routine that follows then you can keep your warm-up shorter. As you begin your warm-up, make sure the intensity is low and increase as you become warmer.

The jumping jacks are great to work on the hip abductors and adductors, calves, everything around the shoulders, and also great to get the blood flowing. The squats work on the ankles, knees, hips, and erector spinae, the hip hinges work on the hamstrings and hip extensors.

If you want to **prepare yourself as best as possible** and work on mind-muscle connection and flexibility as well, then I highly recommend you also perform the *Caveman Kettlebell Swing Muscle Priming Routine* that follows.

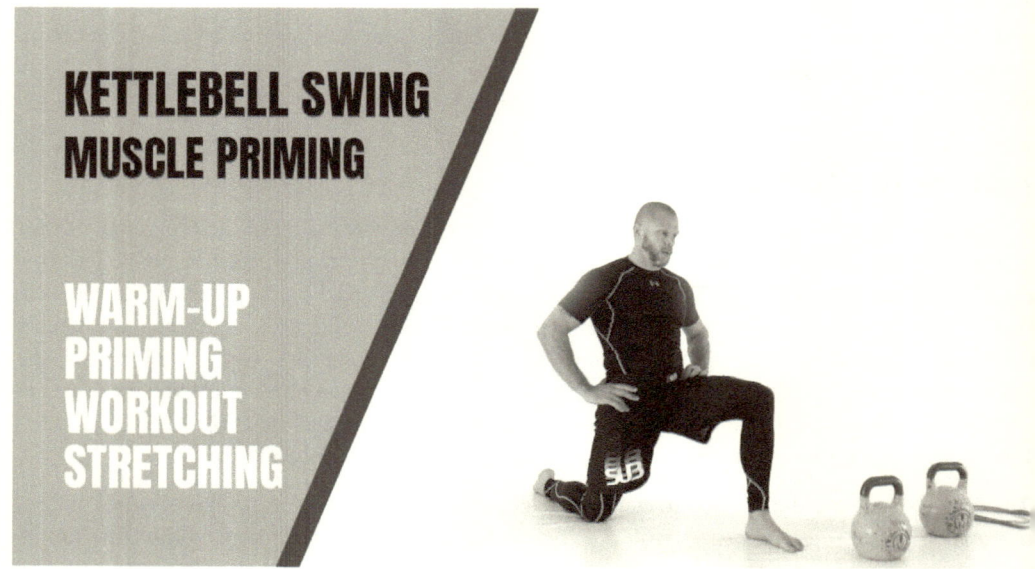

Muscle priming routine

A video for this routine is also included in the bonus material which you can access at the end of this book.

The first part of the routine focuses on getting the hips going, blood flowing, and warming up the body.

- 5 single leg hip circles (each side)
- 10 jumping jacks

Repeat 6 times
Approx. 3 minutes

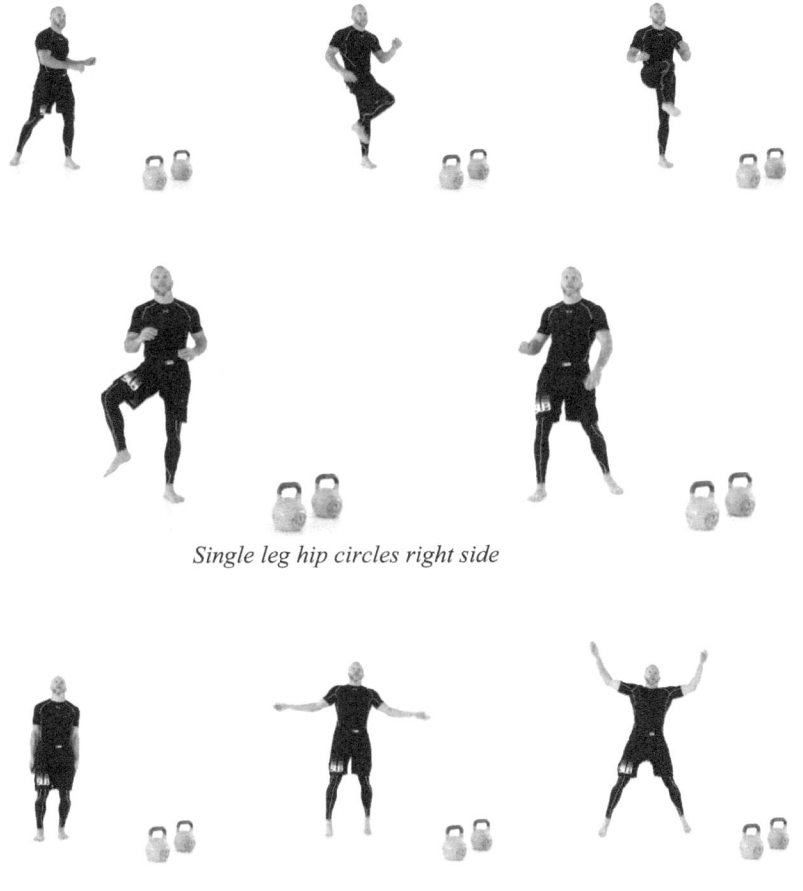

Single leg hip circles right side

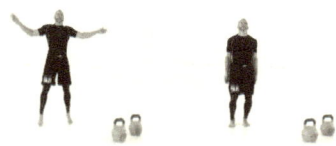

The second part of the warm-up focusses on the hips plus posterior chain.

- Prone hip and thoracic hyperextension into downward dog
- Runners lunge (each side)
- Stand up

Repeat 6 times
Approx. 1 ½ minutes

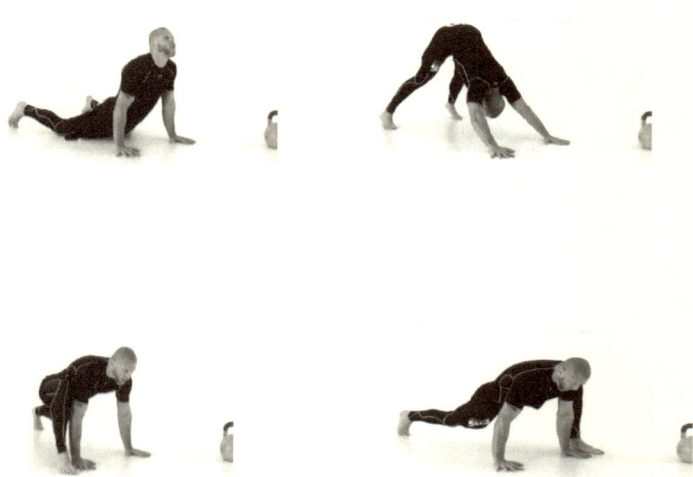

- Prone hip and thoracic hyperextension into downward dog

- Runners lunge and twist (each side)
- Stand up into arms overhead

Repeat 6 times
Approx. 2 minutes

Repeat the warm-up twice.
Approx. 10 minutes

Warning

Hip and thoracic hyperextension should be approached like anything, with progression and care. These two areas are usually not conditioned with the average person, this does not mean it's an area that should not be worked, it means it should be worked and progressed safely. Before you attempt this make sure you understand how to protect your lumbar and create range in with the hips and thoracic.

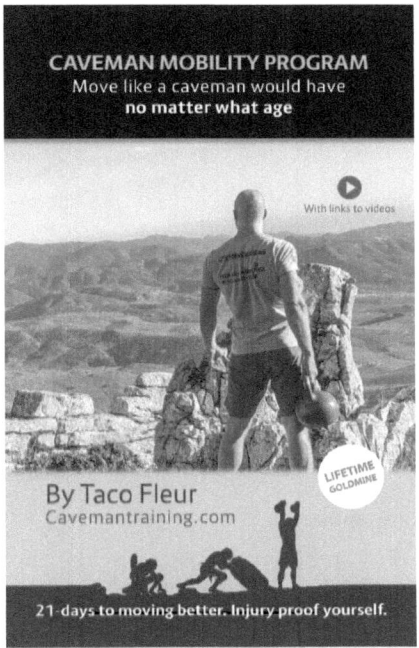

If in doubt, join our free Facebook groups and ask,
or buy the book on Amazon or Cavemantraining.

Muscle priming

This is the part where you're connecting with the areas that are going to do the work for you.

The sequence is as follows:

- 5 x prone single leg hip hyperextensions (each side)
- 5 x prone thoracic hyperextensions
- 5 x kneeling hip extensions
- Kneeling lunge 10 x pulse (each side)
- 5 x true hip hinge
- 5 x quarter squat

Repeat twice
Approx. 4 minutes

Follow up with some shoulder circles to get the upper body loose.

1) Single leg hip hyperextensions

These are to connect with the gluteus maximus and feel the area which is going to do the primary work for you during swings.

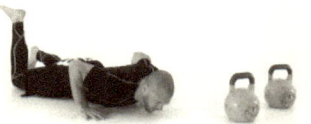 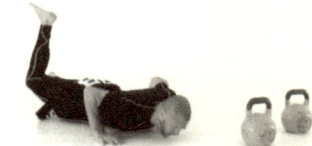

2) Prone thoracic hyperextensions

These are to connect with your erector spinae muscle groups which are to be contracted and simply hold the spine straight (erect) to be moved by the pelvis.

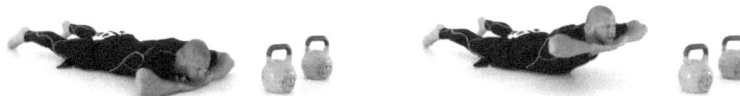

3) Kneeling hip extensions

These are to connect with hamstring muscles which will be pulling at the bottom of your pelvis and help to pull it up during the upswing.

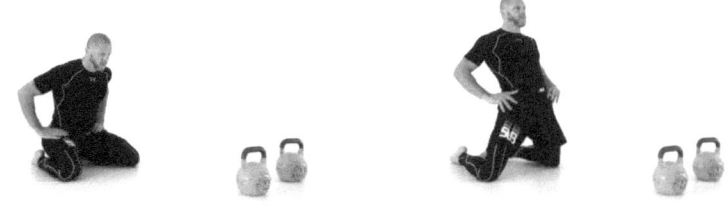

4) Kneeling lunge and pulse

The goals of these is two-fold, the pull with the front leg activates the hamstrings, and the hips coming forward digs into the psoas on the side that the leg is kneeling.

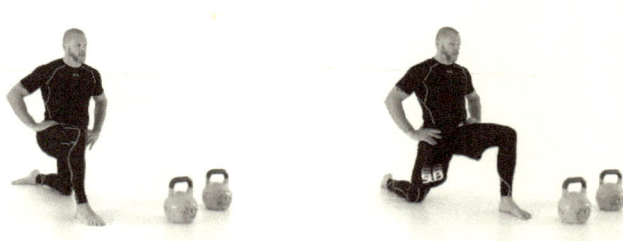

5) True hip hinge

The true hip hinge (AKA stiff-legged hip hinge) prepares you for the primal movement of the kettlebell swing.

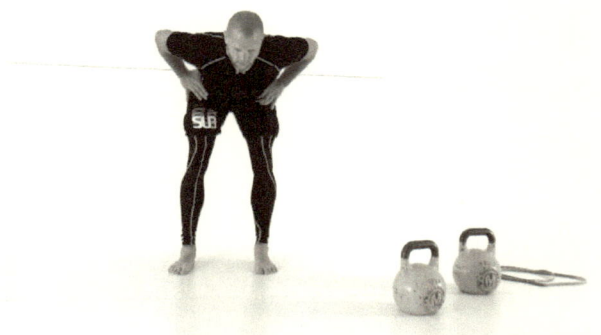

6) Quarter squat

These are to target the quadriceps which are responsible for knee extension which happens at the same time as hip extension.

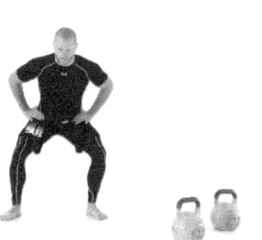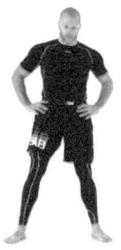

Workout

- 4 x jerk
- 4 x jerk (other side)
- 4 x swings
- 4 x bent-over dead rows
- 4 x bent-over dead rows (other side)
- 4 x swings

4 to 5 rounds or 20 to 30 minutes of work.

The video and other bonus resources can be found at the end of the book.

Frequency

Perform 3 to 5 times a week.

If you're just starting out then you should start with 3 sessions to test the waters, increase to 4 on the following week, and 5 on the subsequent week. If your weight is not heavy enough then you can also increase your sessions to 6 with at least one rest day. Each round should take about 2 to 3 minutes in work and adding about 3 mins for rest in between sets and after a round makes a total of approx 5 to 6 minutes per round. 4 rounds would take about 20 minutes as an average. But investing more time into execution and rest is not going to hurt you but will benefit you.

Progression

Increase reps to 5 in week 3 and 4. Add about 5 minutes if you go by time.

Increase reps to 6 in week 5 and 6. Add about 10 minutes if you go by time.

Take one week off and work on flexibility and mobility or something with light weights.

Repeat the cycle and increase weight or volume.

4 rounds

	Session 1	Session 2	Session 3	Session 4	Session 5
Week 1	4 x 4x6 = 96	4 x 4x6 = 96	4 x 4x6 = 96	4 x 4x6 = 96	4 x 4x6 = 96
Week 2	4 x 4x6 = 96	4 x 4x6 = 96	4 x 4x6 = 96	4 x 4x6 = 96	4 x 4x6 = 96
Week 3	4 x 5x6 = 120	4 x 5x6 = 120	4 x 5x6 = 120	4 x 5x6 = 120	4 x 5x6 = 120
Week 4	4 x 5x6 = 120	4 x 5x6 = 120	4 x 5x6 = 120	4 x 5x6 = 120	4 x 5x6 = 120
Week 5	4 x 6x6 = 144	4 x 6x6 = 144	4 x 6x6 = 144	4 x 6x6 = 144	4 x 6x6 = 144
Week 6	4 x 6x6 = 144	4 x 6x6 = 144	4 x 6x6 = 144	4 x 6x6 = 144	4 x 6x6 = 144
Week 7	Rest				

5 rounds

	Session 1	Session 2	Session 3	Session 4	Session 5
Week 1	5 x 4x6 = 120	5 x 4x6 = 120	5 x 4x6 = 120	5 x 4x6 = 120	5 x 4x6 = 120
Week 2	5 x 4x6 = 120	5 x 4x6 = 120	5 x 4x6 = 120	5 x 4x6 = 120	5 x 4x6 = 120
Week 3	5 x 5x6 = 150	5 x 5x6 = 150	5 x 5x6 = 150	5 x 5x6 = 150	5 x 5x6 = 150
Week 4	5 x 5x6 = 150	5 x 5x6 = 150	5 x 5x6 = 150	5 x 5x6 = 150	5 x 5x6 = 150
Week 5	5 x 6x6 = 180	5 x 6x6 = 180	5 x 6x6 = 180	5 x 6x6 = 180	5 x 6x6 = 180
Week 6	5 x 6x6 = 180	5 x 6x6 = 180	5 x 6x6 = 180	5 x 6x6 = 180	5 x 6x6 = 180
Week 7	Rest				

Rest

Rest after each set, a set is for example 4 swings, or 4 jerks on one side, or 4 rows on one side. Rest longer after a round, a round is when you completed all sets. Include stretching or mobility work in your rest. Depending on how long your rest is after a set you can include some quick dynamic stretching, but after one round you should definitely have enough time to get a good 1 to 3 minutes in.

Rest between workouts should be long enough to be able to recover enough to go into each workout with the same vigor as you came and attacked your very first session. If you feel that you're lacking the energy then you should program more rest and recovery. Rest and recovery means:

- good and enough sleep
- good and healthy food
- no other strenuous tasks

If you are too sore to train you need to increase your rest or reduce the weight. You can also reduce the rounds until you feel that your recovery is getting much better and you feel as vigorous as when you started. Look at including more anti-inflammatory ingredients in your nutrition, try cold showers, epsom salt baths, foam roll, and above all, keep moving. Movement in my opinion is going to be the best out of all, but not intense movement, or loaded movement, focus on slow movements to increase range and keep it dynamic but slow. Great time to work on your mobility.

Accountability

We all know how easy it is to start something and not finish it. Get accountable, post on your Facebook or in our groups today that you're starting the *Prometheus Kettlebell Strength Program.*

Hashtag: #cavemantraining
Instagram: @realcavemantraining
Facebook: @Cavemantraining
Reddit: u/cavemankettlebells or r/Kettlebell_training

Post in one of our kettlebell groups.

Kettlebell Training 10,000 members https://www.facebook.com/groups/KettlebellTraining
Kettlebell Enthusiasts 2,400 members https://www.facebook.com/groups/kettlebell.enthusiasts
Kettlebell Workouts 2,000 members https://www.facebook.com/groups/kettlebell.workout
Caveman Inner Circle **PRIVATE** https://www.facebook.com/groups/caveman.inner.circle/

Exercise selection

The exercises were carefully chosen for the following reasons. The first goal was to keep the exercise selection to a minimum. Both the swing and jerk are a full-body exercise, the swings hit the full posterior chain and quads, the jerks hit the legs and arms, and the rows work the upper part of the back which is usually neglected in training. All this combined will require recruitment of just about every muscle in your body. How much of them you hit also depends on how well you contract everything and how well you connect with everything.

Kettlebell jerks

The focus of the jerk is the quadriceps, gluteus maximus, biceps femoris (long head), semitendinosus, semimembranosus, adductor magnus, triceps brachii, anconeus, deltoid, serratus anterior, coracobrachialis, and biceps brachii.

The kettlebell jerk is a push press and then dip under with elbow fully extended and the arm positioned overhead. Another way to describe this is a double-dip, the first one is to launch the weight up, the second one is to come under, and then you stand up. The jerk is an advanced movement. Proper racking is important for a good jerk. A jerk requires a clean, a clean requires a good insert and grip, download the free kettlebell grips PDF (see resources at the end of book).

Push press

The push press is half powered by the legs and half by the shoulder(s). From racking the knees flex and rapidly extend while driving into and keeping the heels on the floor. The push press is the progression to the jerk. On that note, the jerk is not a press, after the push with the legs you would come under the weight rather than pressing out as you would with the push press.

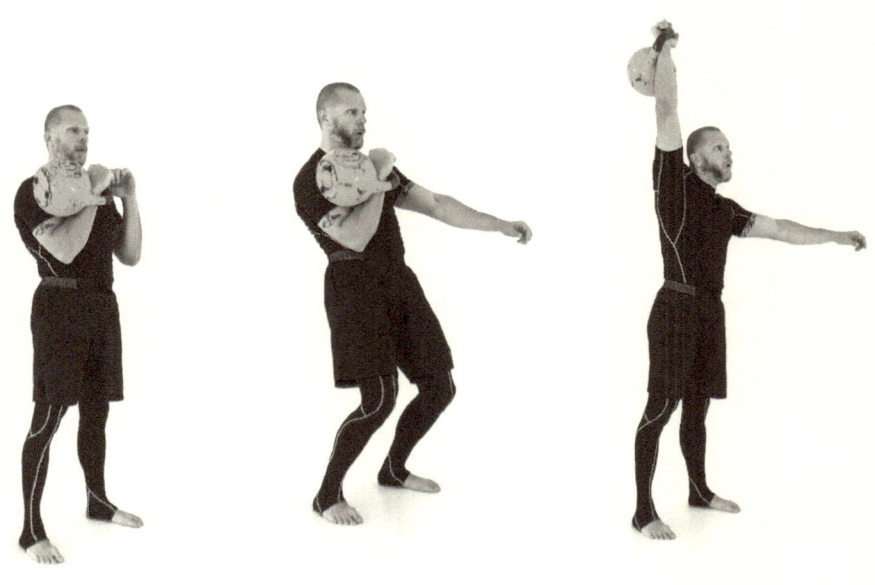

Jerk

The first part of the jerk is a push press that's not pressed out. Immediately after the push there is the second dip which is to come under the weight (photo 3) with the arm locked out. From there the next position is coming into full extension with the arm still overhead. The weight is then dropped into rack and another jerk is performed.

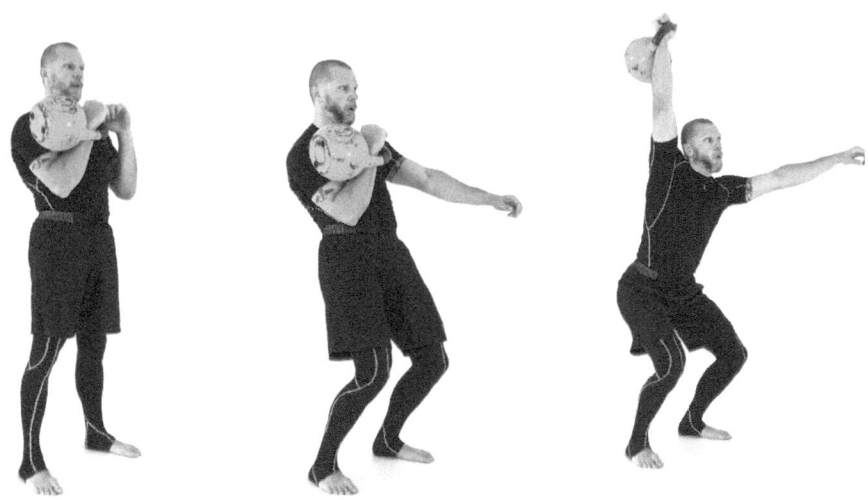

Key safety point to consider. When you're in the under squat you should pay great attention to the alignment of your pelvis. The pelvis should be aligned with your spine, you control this alignment with your gluteus maximus, i.e. through contraction which pulls the pelvis back in line with the spine.

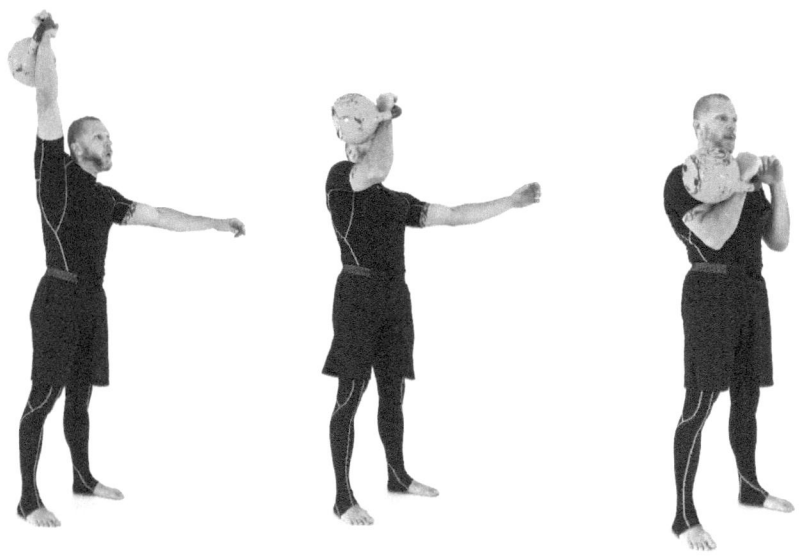

The easiest way to think about the jerk is to push your knees forward and back immediately, this is to push the weight up, then you drop your hips low to come under the weight and push yourself away from the weight. There is no pressing in the jerk. Once you're under the weight and everything is solid and not moving you come up out of the under squat after which you keep the weight overhead for a split second without movement.

A good rack is important for a good jerk. Racking is something that sounds so simple yet during my career I have found it one of the most difficult things for athletes to grasp, so I'm going to devote quite some information to it and I will do so from a generic perspective, i.e. not just for the jerk and not just for single kettlebell work as only is required for this program. As you progress you will want to work with double bells and this information will also lay that groundwork for you.

Bent-over dead rows

The focus of the bent-over row is the rear delt, latissimus dorsi, teres major, and triceps brachii (long head), but there is way more going on as you create a stable base to row/pull the heavyweight from. You lunge forward and take a step back to create the position to row from. Your back remains neutral and your non-working arm is resting on the forward knee. Make sure you row and aren't performing bicep curls, if you find that the weight is not moving back and up but remains under and toward the shoulder then you're bicep curling.

Key safety point to consider. When you first start rowing there is a progression of flexibility that needs to be followed. Your shoulder extension does not have to exaggerated, it's quite common for people to really want to pull that weight high as the range doesn't feel like a lot. Slowly progress, yes, the higher you come the more range you get but it should not be at the expense of injury, if you have limited range then holding and pausing at a safe range will also get you that time under tension.

Bent-over rows

The bent-over rows are performed as per following photo.

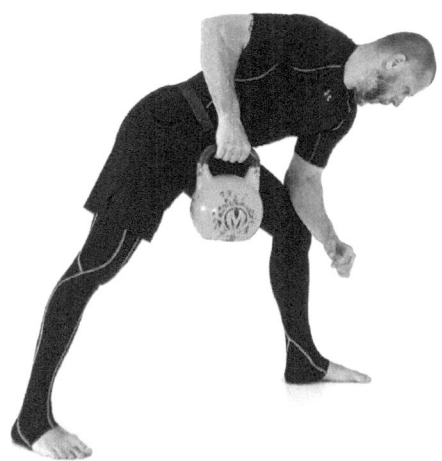

You can perform them as shown in the next sequence which allows you to put your weight on the kettlebell through the non-working arm.

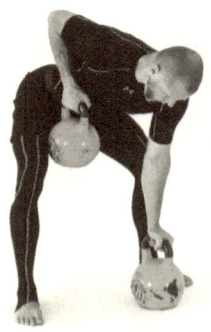 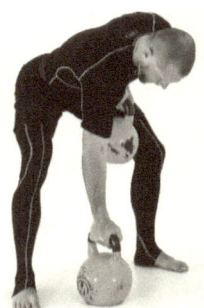

If it feel better, you can also put your feet closer together and row on the outside of the legs as demonstrated in the following sequence of photos.

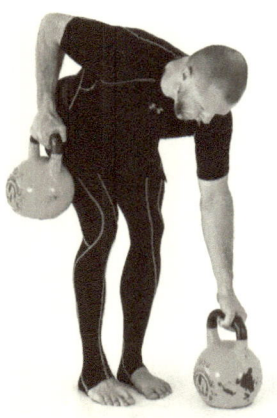 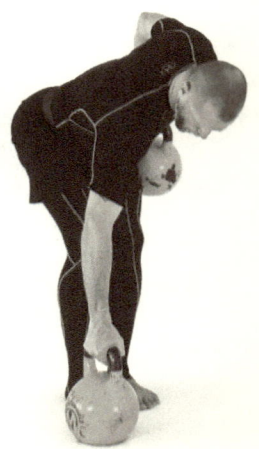

Kettlebell swings

The kettlebell swings are performed with a hip hinge which means you prevent movement in your ankles, there is flexion and extension in the knees and hips. A full step-by-step description of the movement is further down.

Key safety point to consider. Don't follow the kettlebell, protect the lower back! A video about this is included in the bonus material that you can view online. At the top of the swing when the kettlebell is going back down you do not want to follow it and break at the hips the same time the kettlebell goes back down, this will put a lot of pressure on the lower back, instead, wait for the kettlebell to be at a good height to create hip flexion and keep the back safe. A good height is usually when the bell is or nears the legs.

The kettlebell swing is a full-body exercise that uses muscles for grip, posture, stabilization, to keep the spine erect, and the actual movement (prime movers). I cover the two-handed swing, the single-handed swing would involve a lot more action around the mid-section.

Grip

- Flexor digitorum superficialis
- Flexor digitorum profundus
- Flexor digit minimi brevis
- Lumbricals

Posture/shoulders

- Rhomboideus minor
- Rhomboideus major
- Lower trapezius
- Levator scapulae
- Latissimus dorsi

Spine

- Iliocostalis
- Longissimus
- Spinalis

Prime movers

- Gluteus maximus
- Bicep femoris (long head)
- Semitendinosus
- Semimembranosus

Flexion and stabilization

- Biceps femoris
- Semitendinosus
- Semimembranosus
- Gracilis
- Sartorius
- Gastrocnemius
- Soleus
- Popliteus

Grip

The muscles used for grip are usually not mentioned or thought off, however, your swing is only as good as your grip. In fact, most of your training is only as good as your grip, if you have a weak grip then you won't be lifting heavy. If your grip has no endurance then you won't be completing high reps unbroken.

Posture/shoulders

I'm referring to the top part of your body at the top of the swing where your shoulders are nice and safely pulled down. Your chest it out, shoulders blades slightly down and pulled together.

Spine

Throughout the swing, your erector spinae muscles need to work to keep your spine erect, and there is actually a lot more going on inside as well to protect the spine and brace the abs.

Prime movers

These are the muscles that create the movement which is the hip and knee extension only when we're talking about the conventional kettlebell swing.

Flexion and stabilization

The flexion I refer to is knee flexion and the stabilization I refer to is that of keeping the knee in place above the ankle. Keeping the knee above the ankle is important when hip hinging, if the knee comes excessively forward, then the movement starts to turn into a squat. A kettlebell squat swing is not bad, it's only bad if you need to perform a hip hinge and perform a squat, or perform the squat swing incorrectly, otherwise, the squat swing is an excellent exercise. See a side by side comparison of the hip hinge versus squat swing.

Double arm

AKA Russian swing, conventional swing.

Conventional: Based on or in accordance with what is generally done or believed.

It should be noted that although this is referred to as the conventional swing, this is only due to this movement is what popularized the kettlebell swing and is the most common variation of the swing seen outside of sport. If you'd wanted to look at this from the perspective of what variation of the swing came first then it would be the pendulum swing from kettlebell sport, which was used in Russia way before the kettlebell swing became popular outside of Russia.

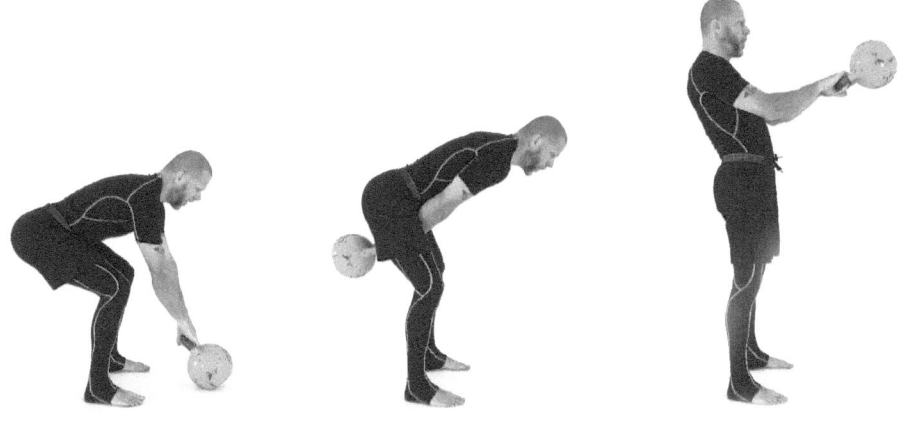

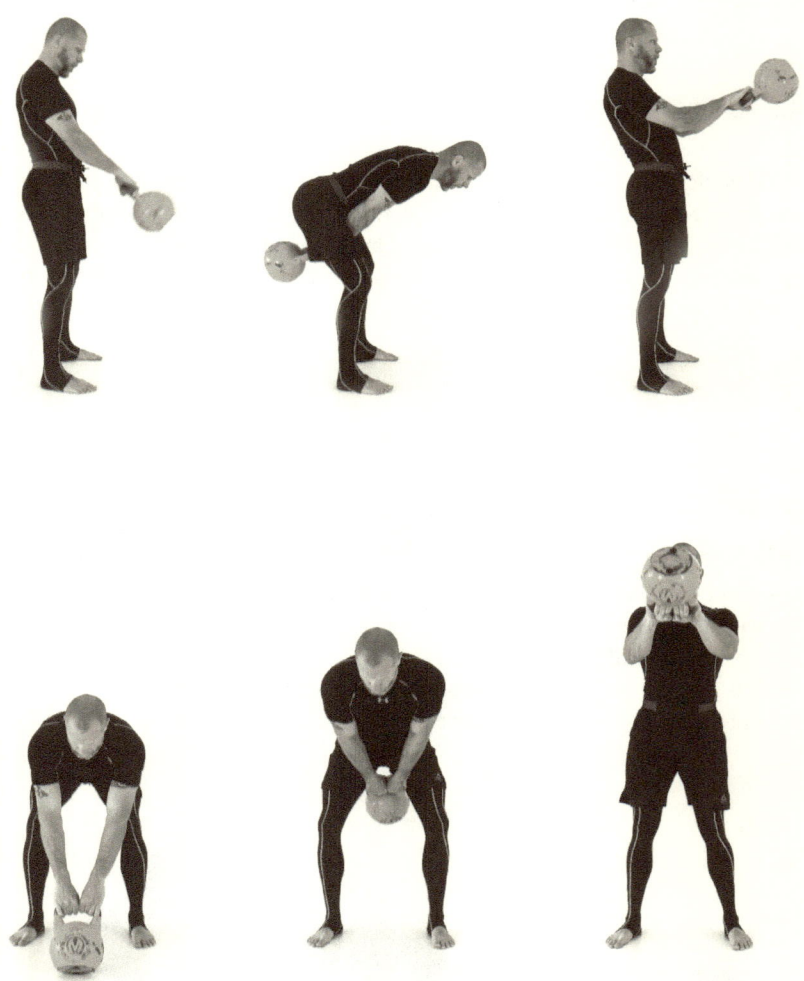

Prometheus Strength Program Taco Fleur

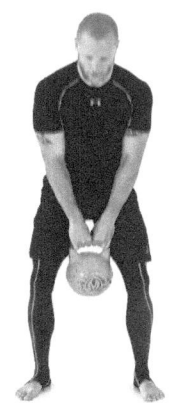 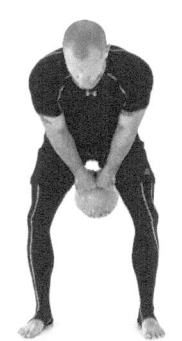 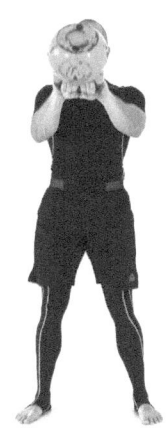

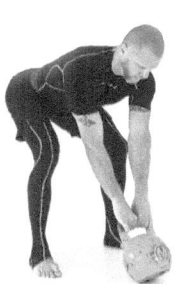 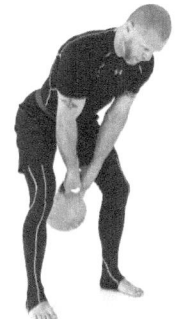 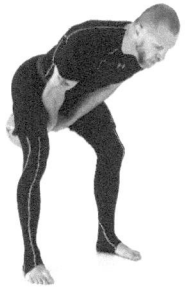

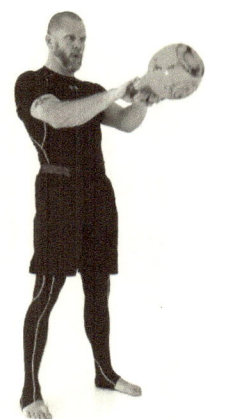 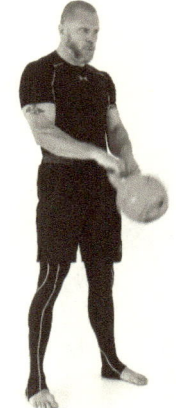 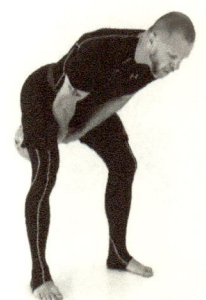

To perform the double arm swing with one kettlebell:

1. **START OF THE SWING** Stand in a neutral position

2. Feet slightly wider than shoulder-width

3. Kettlebell placed in-front of you

4. Maintain a neutral spine and braced core

5. Maintain flat feet on the ground

6. Maintain straight arms
   (this can change once you've mastered the swing)

7. Maintain relaxed shoulders

8. Think of the arms as a rod and shoulders as a pivot

9. Hip hinge and reach for the kettlebell
   (do not overreach)

10. Grab the kettlebell by the handle with both hands and a loose grip

11. Create slight tension between yourself and the kettlebell

12. Pull the kettlebell off the ground and hike it back through the legs

13. <u>Slightly</u> bring the shoulders up during the pull from the ground and into the back swing

14. The height at which the kettlebell comes through should be around knee height

15. Elbows making connection with the belly around the first ribs of the ribcage

16. The outside of the wrist making connection or being around the inside thigh area

17. Direct the kettlebell to the back

18. **UPSWING** Initiate the pull out

19. Press the heels into the ground with weight evenly distributed across the foot

20. Contract the gluteus maximus to pull the pelvis up and propel the bell forward

21. Contract the hamstring muscles to assist in pulling the pelvis up

22. Follow through with an explosive but controlled full hip extension

23. Full knee extension

24. The whole body comes into extension

25. The power from the lower-body; and the upper-body coming upright is what propels the kettlebell

26. Do not lean back at the lumbar to pull the weight higher
(proper hip hyper extension is different and might be required when working with heavy weights to create counterbalance)

27. **FLOAT**
The top of the swing is when the kettlebell is motionless in the air for a split second

28. The kettlebell only needs to swing as high as the force generated by your lower-body will move it; which is usually about chest height

29. At the top of the swing remember:

   ☐ Chest out

   ☐ Shoulders back

   ☐ Latissimus dorsi pulled down

- ☐ Core braced

- ☐ Gluteals squeezed

- ☐ Legs are straight

- ☐ Look ahead

30. **BACKSWING** Get ready to break at the hips when the kettlebell starts to fall down

31. Delay breaking of the hips as long as possible to prevent unbalancing the movement
(the heavier the weight or the more fatigue is present the longer the delay)

32. The kettlebell should come through the legs approximately around the knees
(you should be able to put another kettlebell between your legs and not hit it)

33. Perform an insert and push the weight through

34. Elbows/forearms should be making contact around the waist line

35. You should feel tension on the hamstrings when pushing the hips back

36. Remember that **this version** of the swing is not a squat

37. **REPEAT UPSWING**

The hip hinge
- hip flexion paired with knee flexion
- hips moving back and slightly down
- knees remain positioned above the ankles/shins vertical
- no ankle dorsiflexion
- shoulders come toward the ground
- approximately 45 to 60 degrees of flexion in the hips and knees
- followed by extension in the hips and knees
- coming into full extension

Breathing
You can inhale on the down-phase and exhale on the up-phase. You can inhale through the nose and out through the mouth or do both through the mouth. You can forcefully breathe out through the mouth when up or down, the inhale happens automatically during the movement. Whatever breathing pattern you choose, do not hold your breath during the swing.

Single arm swing

If you have one kettlebell that is not as heavy as it should be for this program then you can switch the double arm swing to single arm and double the set, i.e. 4 double arm swings becomes 4 single arm swings on each side (8 in total). There still is a minimum for this change to be effective, i.e. if you should be swinging a 48kg/105lb double arm but only have a 12kg/26lb then the weight is simply too light as you'll want something that is at least half the weight, i.e. 24kg/53lb and up, but even 20kg/44lb would be ok and just increase the reps by 2 or 4.

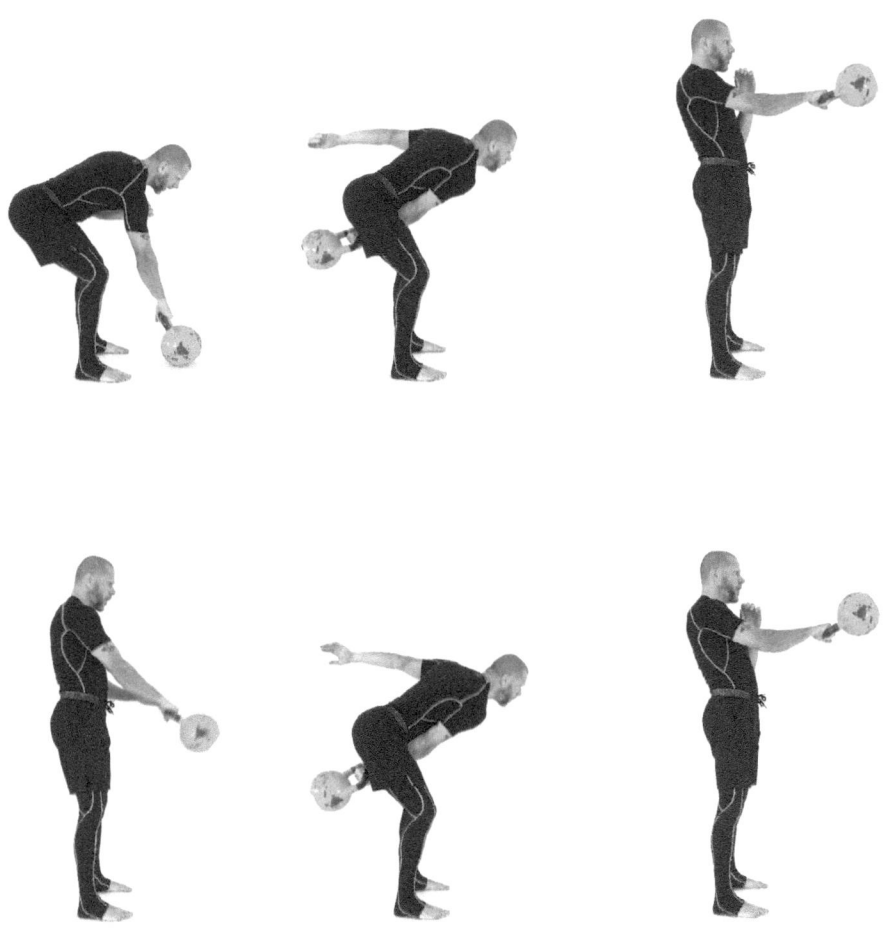

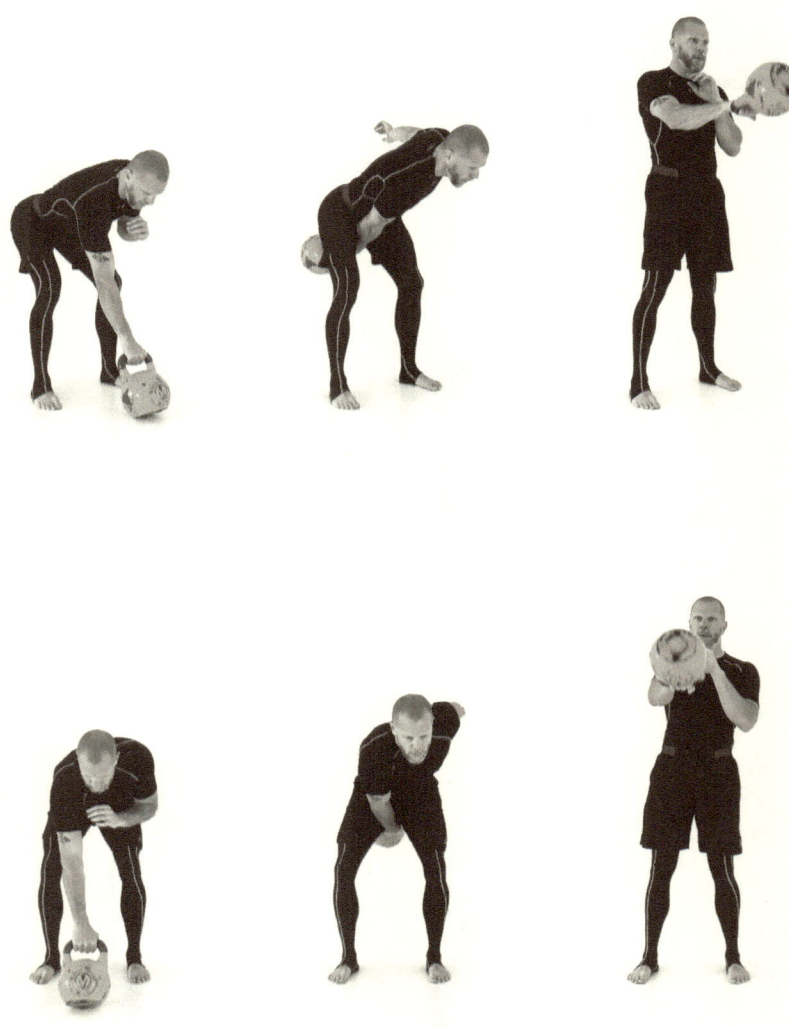

Double kettlebell

If you don't have one heavy kettlebell but you have two kettlebells, then you can do double kettlebell swings. Even if the weights were uneven you can replace the single kettlebell swing for double. The recommended weight difference should be no more than 4 or 8kg but you can test. When you do work with two different weight kettlebells you need to make sure to switch on sets.

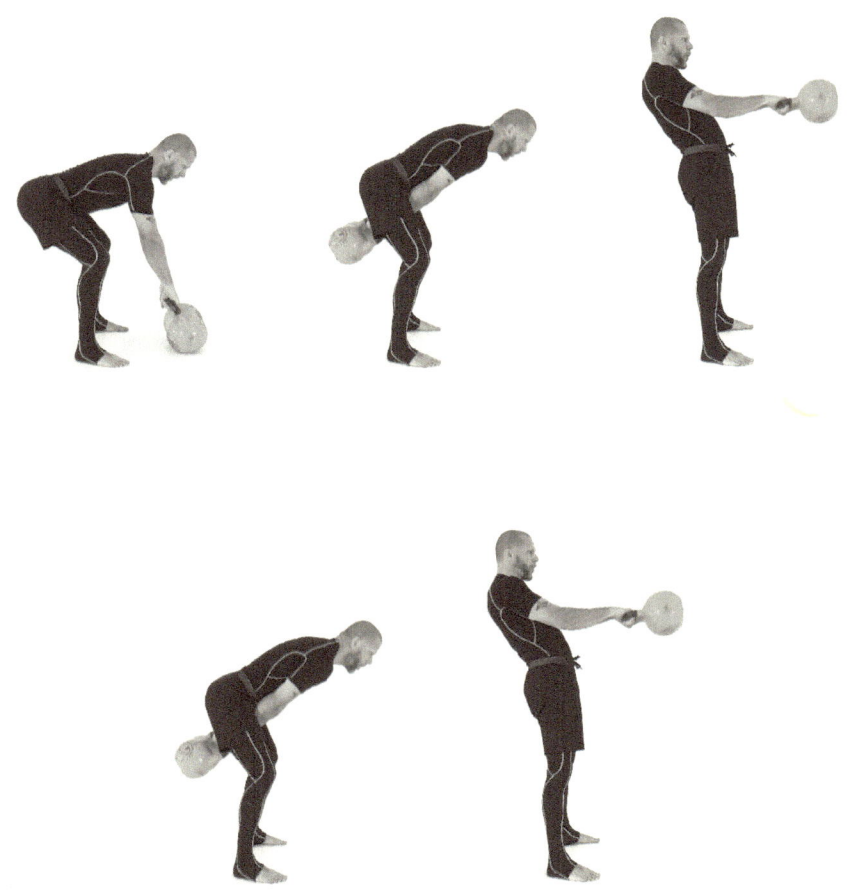

The following two photos displays the differences between handle angles. The first photo is a swing with a 90 degree handle angle which turns the thumb up and elbow down.

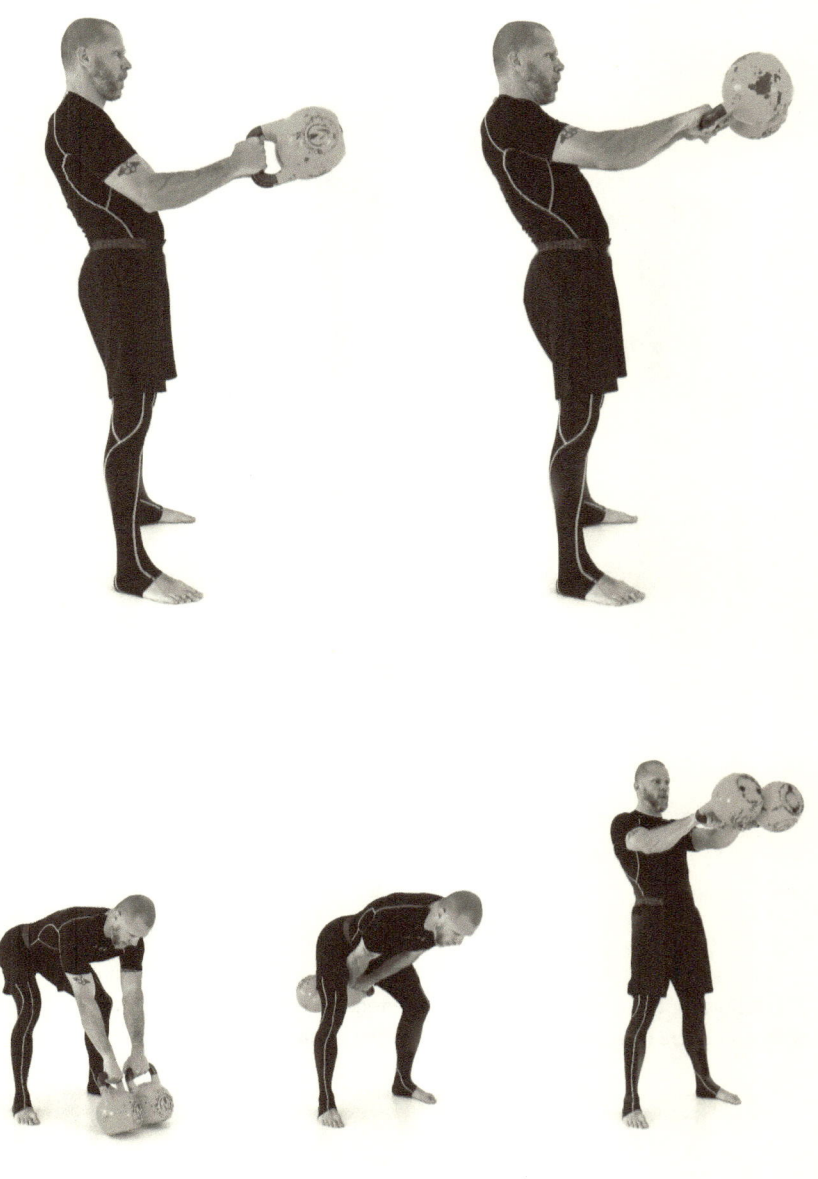

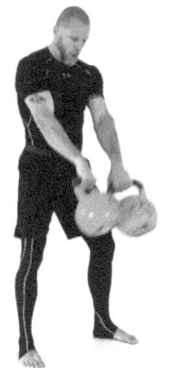 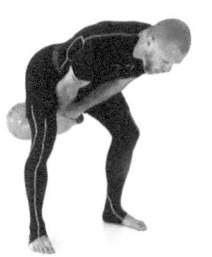 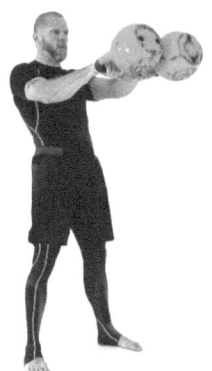

Squat swing

As you go extremely heavy you'll find it becomes harder to prevent dorsiflexion in the ankles which will turn this into a squat and that's not necessarily a bad thing. Do your best to avoid it. Sometimes you might even want to mix it up as you're including more quads work and taking pressure of the lower back. So, it's great to mix it up but also if you feel a tingle in your lower back for some reason, that feeling where you know there is something not 100% but it's not something that requires you to stop.

The kettlebell swing squat style is performed in similar fashion to the conventional swing, with the following differences:

1. Four joints involved rather than three

2. The upper-body remains more vertical during the swing

3. The shins no longer remain vertical during the swing and come forward

4. Ankle dorsiflexion is created

5. The trajectory of the swing is down and up rather than forward and back

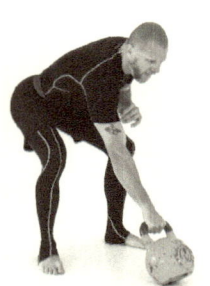 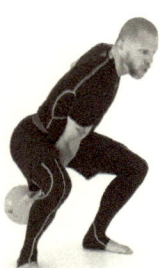 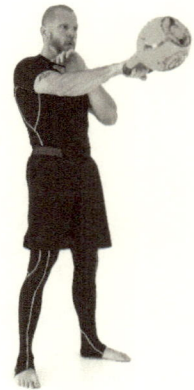

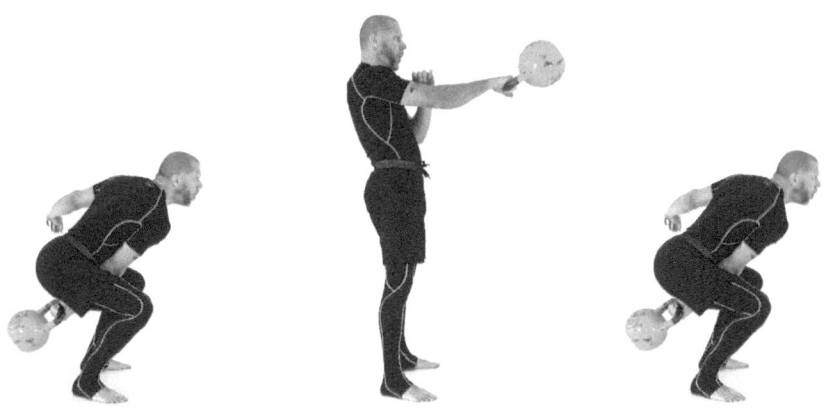

The following two photos display the clear differences between a squat and hip hinge swing. In the first photo there is a clear ankle dorsiflexion (knees coming forward), the hips are lower, and the torso is more upright.

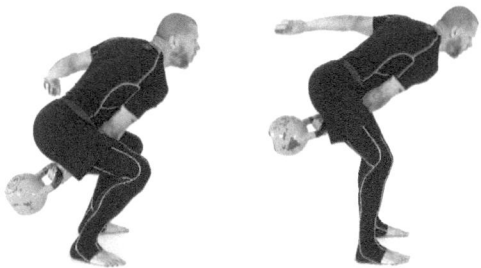

Double arm

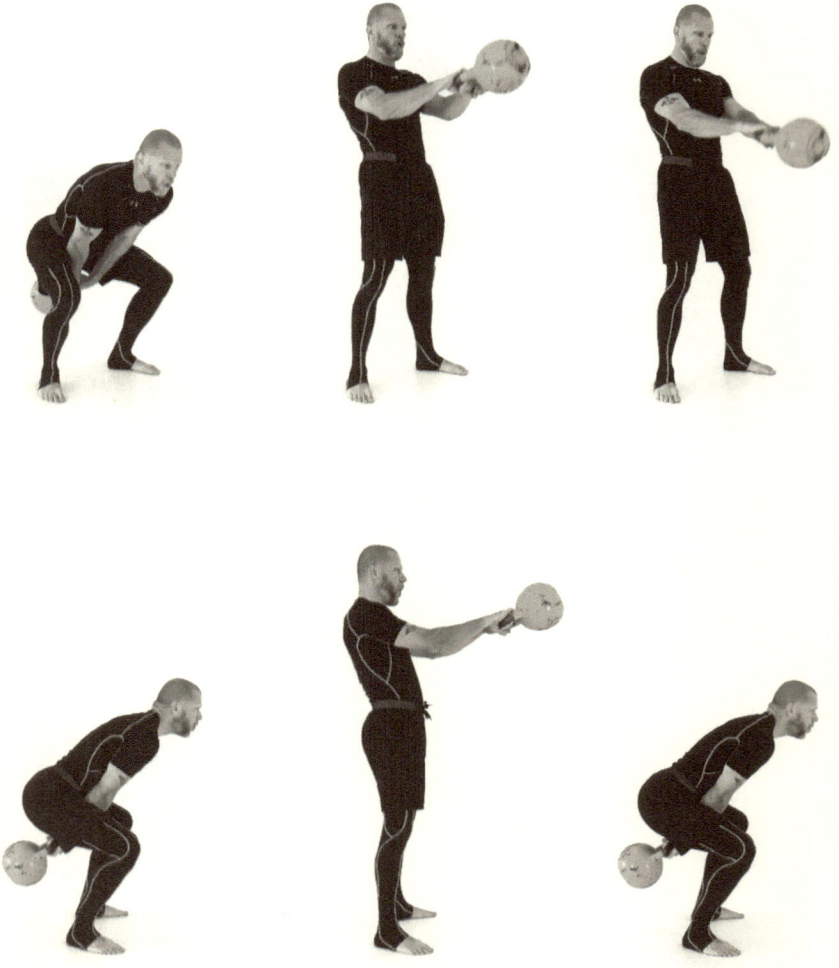

Racking

Why rack properly?

The <u>main</u> points why you should rack your kettlebell properly are:

- Conserve energy
- Be able to rest when required
- Allow for proper power transfer
- Avoid injury

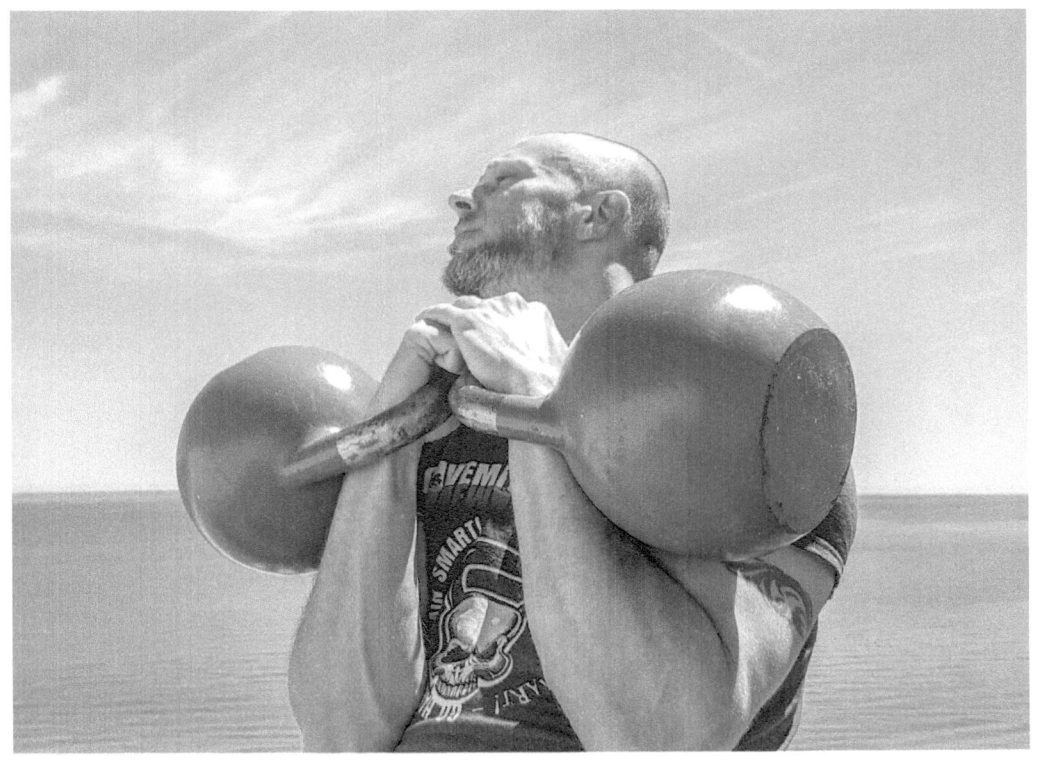

Conserve energy to last longer in sets by being able to relax the muscles more when in proper racking position.

Being able to **rest** when required, i.e. when doing high volume reps, and not having to put the kettlebells down, as this would require more energy and time.

Properly transfer power when doing jerks or push presses; transfer the power from the legs directly into the forearm through the elbow, rather than directing and losing power through the torso, shoulders, and elbows.

Avoid injury by removing stress on the shoulders joints or muscles.

Common Grips in Racking

Following are the common grips used in the racking position:

- Racking grip

- Racking safety grip

- Flat hand grip

- Interlocking grip

- Stacking grip

For more details on all kettlebell grips available, download our free PDF with over 25+ kettlebell grips. Search Google for '*Cavemantraining Kettlebell Grips*'.

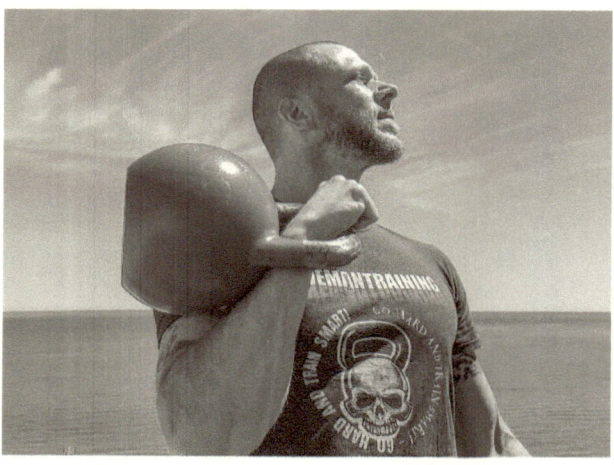

See the clean and rack in action. 300 unbroken clean and jerks with a 20kg/44lb kettlebell
go.cavemantraining.com/mkr-vid3

Racking Points and Tips

Following are some points and tips that I'm able to help my students find their <u>one bell racking position</u> easily.

The first step is to find the racking position without weight, using the following moves and cues to practice the one bell racking position.

Bodyweight practice

1. Stand straight in a neutral position
2. Bend one arm to bring the hand to the chest
3. Keep the elbow tucked in
4. Loosen the hips
5. Squeeze the gluteus maximus to pull the top of the pelvis back (hip hyperextension)
6. Move the top of the femurs slightly forward (ankle dorsiflexion)
7. Fill the chest with a deep breath of air
8. Release all the air while crunching forward (thoracic flexion)
9. Crunch to the side (thoracic lateral flexion)
10. Push the hip slightly towards the side on which you're racking

Make adjustments if the forearm is not directly vertically aligned with the leg.

Spine

The upper part of the torso needs to come away from its natural position, which, in a neutral standing position would be in line with the hips. Why? Consider your body being in a normal neutral standing position while racking two heavy kettlebells, all the weight would be pulling you forward, this would keep the body under tension, wear out the biceps, and provide you with no rest. *See the infographic below.*

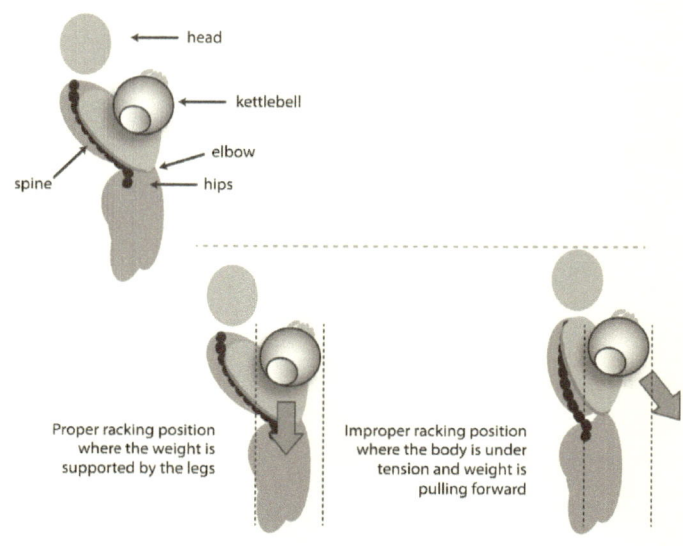

Now consider the spine making space for the kettlebells, allowing the weight to be placed above the hips, and supported by the legs. *See the infographic below.*

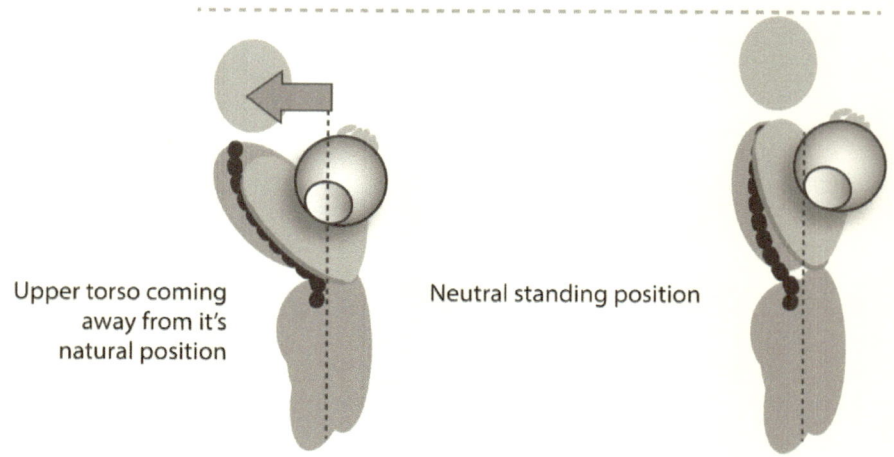

What is hip (hyper)extension?

Our definition for hyperextension is most likely different from other writings. Following is the explanation of hyperextension under the context of Cavemantraining material.

Hip flexion is where you pull the top of the pelvis down towards the ground, and extension is the opposite. Hip hyperextension is not something everyone can do right away, you need flexibility at the front, something you'll need to work on over time.

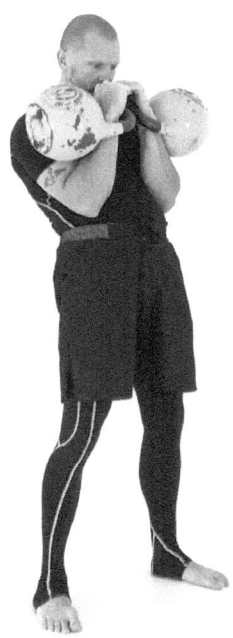

In a neutral position you'd be in extension, going further back, i.e. pulling the pelvis further back, is called hip hyperextension. But most people associate 'injury' with the word *hyperextension*, and its definition is:

> *Hyperextension is an excessive joint movement in which the angle formed by the bones of a particular joint is opened, or straightened, beyond its normal, healthy, range of motion.*

> *Hyper means: over; beyond; above.*

Hyperextension without flexibility is indeed a cause for injury. Hyperextension in joints that are not made to hyperextend is also cause for injury. Hyperextension with proper flexibility and progression is something everyone should strive for. Joints that can be hyperextended through proper progression:

- Hips
- Spine (back/neck)

You create hip extension by squeezing the gluteus maximus and letting the top of the femur come slightly forward, i.e. normally positioned above the ankles, now coming forward towards the toes. This action tilts the pelvis backward. On top of the pelvis is the spine, this follows along naturally—looking like back hyperextension—if you keep it positioned neutrally.

The second step is to crunch, bring the shoulders and head forward, this is done via thoracic flexion, the same action you make when performing crunches on the ground.

Racking should not be confused with back hyperextension, although back hyperextensions are also something one should be doing, and is completely safe with proper progression, it's not a safe nor an efficient position to rest in with heavy weights.

Back hyperextension is actually the complete opposite of what a good racking position is. A good racking position is thoracic flexion (think crunching), hip hyperextension, with knee extension, and slight ankle dorsiflexion.

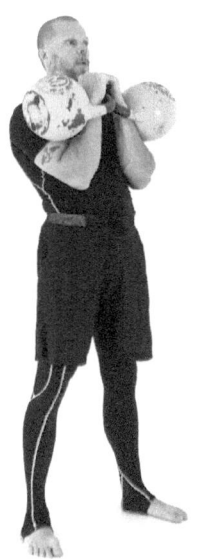 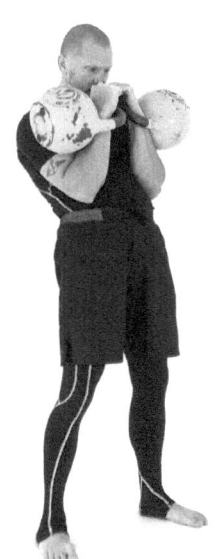

Racking Cues

Following are racking cues you can use, for yourself, or to help a student find a proper racking position:

- The hips are soft and not locked
- Elbow is resting on the hip/ilium or as close as possible
- Straight wrist if the bell is resting on the forearm
- Slightly bend wrist when the bell is resting between forearm and biceps
- Handle at a 45-degree angle within the palm
- Loose grip
- Relax your shoulders and upper trapezius
- Round the back (thoracic flexion)
- Think about creating a side-on 'S' shape with your body
- The forearm should not hurt with proper weight distribution
- The space for the kettlebell is **not** created by lower back hyper extension

Kettlebell resting position

The kettlebell can rest on the forearm or between the forearm and biceps, this is determined by the angle between the hand and the chest, if the hand is more towards the chest, the bell will be resting more on the forearm, if the hand comes more away from the chest—increasing the angle—then the bell will be resting more between the forearm and biceps. Women with larger breasts will need to rest the kettlebell between the forearm and biceps plus increase the angle.

Most trainers recommend to lock the knees out (legs straight), which makes sense, let the weight rest on the skeletal system and not the muscles. I find this doesn't always work for everyone and more comfortable positions can be found with the knees slightly bent. Knees slightly bent also helps if you're not very flexible at the hips, this allows you to move the weight above the feet without great hip flexibility. Use what works best for you.

Flexibility

When there is a lack of flexibility in the hips, it's quite alright to create the angles required through slight knee flexion (bending the knees). However, the objective is to work on hip flexibility, as bending the knees requires more quadriceps work.

The racking concept

In the end, it's about understanding the main concepts of racking, do what you can to get the maximum benefit from these concepts and you're doing good.

- Let the skeletal system take as much of the weight as possible
- Let your legs do the work

If you're not meeting those points you can experience fatigue in the shoulders and biceps. The shoulders will be affected because your arms are disconnected, the biceps—or rather all elbow flexors—will be affected because the weight is not resting on the skeletal system.

With all that said, it should be known that there is not one position for all, every body is different, adjustments need to be made accordingly, and some people just won't be able to get a perfect racking position. Some might need to employ **a racking position with a** <u>stacking grip</u> **and rest on one hip by leaning off to one side. In the end, a**s long as the effort is made and the points are understood you should be good.

If you can't obtain a good racking position no matter what, then you should consider resting in overhead lock-out.

Racking positions explained

The straight standing racking position is the one in which you transition to another exercise like the strict shoulder press, military press, half snatch, or another clean. There is no need to obtain a resting rack or rack to transfer power from the legs, hence, there is no need to waste time on creating hip and thoracic hyperextension to get the elbows to the ilium.

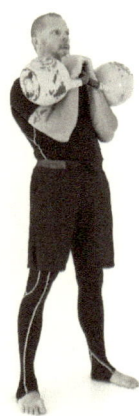

The racking position in which you take the effort to get the elbows to the ilium is the position from which you transition into a jerk or push press, or rest. A resting position is used in endurance work.

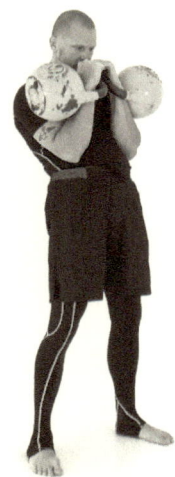

These photos are part of a 5,000+ large kettlebell exercise library owned by Cavemantraining and you'll find our photos in our courses, apps, or books.

The cradle racking position is a position that is employed by women, but also men for many different reasons to increase efficiency, reduce rotation, and more, but this is getting advanced.

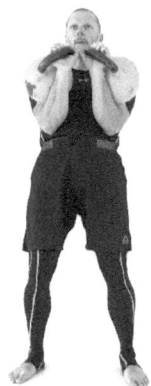 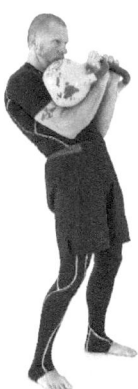

The racking position with interlocking grip is another grip for resting, but can also be used for front squats. Use it especially if you're having trouble with the kettlebells coming apart.

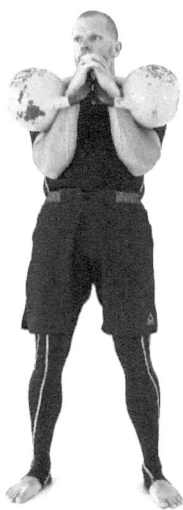

If this short section opened up a world of kettlebell information to you, I can highly recommend checking out our free kettlebell grips book. Knowing kettlebell grips will help avoid injury, can make you more efficient, and can spice up your training. Grip PDF go.cavemantraining.com/mkr-link2

The racking position with flat hand grip is one I like to implement sometimes when doing jerks, it allows me to rest the hands and keep the fingers safe. When doing high volume it does matter whether you close your hands every time or not. Again, this is also a great grip if you've got your fingers caught between the handles before.

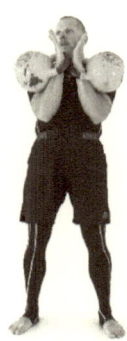

The following is what I like to call the disconnected rack, this is a racking position mostly seen with beginners. This position puts a lot of strain on the shoulders as they remain in flexion the whole time.

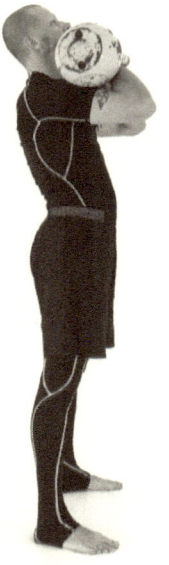 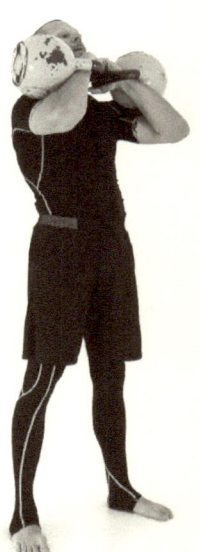

This short section on racking truly just scratches the surface of the information that we've compiled on kettlebell training over the last decade. Kettlebell training is amazing, kettlebell training can provide amazing results in many different areas, cardio, strength, agility, flexibility, endurance, and so on. But, the kettlebell comes with a much higher learning curve than most other exercise tools, if you respect that and invest the time in it, it will pay you high dividends.

Racking problems

Following are a few of the common problems that can occur with racking and make kettlebells unpleasant.

Elbow flexors: Biceps brachii, brachioradialis, and brachialis
Possible cause: The weight is not directly supported above the legs, is falling forward, and requiring elbow flexion (think bicep curling).

Chest: Pectoralis major
Possible cause: The weight is not directly supported above the legs, is falling laterally, and requiring shoulder medial rotation. Also see arm/elbow disconnection below.

Shoulders: Anterior deltoid
Possible cause: The arm(s)/elbow(s) are disconnected from the body/hip(s), the weight needs to be supported by the shoulders, and requiring shoulder flexion.

Resources:

- Kettlebell Workouts and Challenges 1.0 book
- Kettlebell Workouts and Challenges 2.0 book
- Master Kettlebell Grips PDF

Bonus resources

The video and other bonus resources can be accessed on the following link with the password **X8QKHMUN** www.cavemantraining.com/prometheus

For those that feel like they're missing the foundations of kettlebell training or want to get better at kettlebell training Cavemantraining is providing huge discounts below to courses that I know will take you to that next level. Valid for purchasers of this book only.

The **kettlebell training for beginners** course is directly related to this book as it will teach you all the fundamentals of kettlebell training, swing, press, clean, row, etc. **HIGHLY RECOMMENDED**

www.udemy.com/kettlebell-training-for-beginners/?couponCode=BLJCYTZZ
Coupon code BLJCYTZZ   *Normally $74.99 but $9.99 with coupon*

The **kettlebell clean** course is directly related to this book as you need to clean your kettlebell for your jerk. This course will teach you how to clean and prevent common injuries and annoyances. **HIGHLY RECOMMENDED**

www.udemy.com/kettlebell-exercise/?couponCode=E8FJE3VZ
Coupon code E8FJE3VZ   *Normally $79.99 but $9.99 with coupon*

The **kettlebell press** course is directly related to this book as it's a strength exercise and also is going to improve your overhead work for the jerk.

www.udemy.com/kettlebells-for-shoulder-strength/?couponCode=YRVOND43
Coupon code YRVOND43   *Normally $39.99 but $9.99 with coupon*

The **CAVEMANROM kettlebells for flexibility and mobility** is related to this course as increased mobility and flexibility is going to keep you safer and make you stronger in the long in the long run.

www.udemy.com/kettlebells-for-mobility/?couponCode=E7ZJUSTF
Coupon code E7ZJUSTF   *Normally $199.99 but $19.99 with coupon*

The **kettlebell snatch** course is not directly related to this book but is not for nothing called the king of kettlebell exercises, hence an exercise which provides countless benefits.

www.udemy.com/kettlebell-snatch/?couponCode=SUH3RELX
Coupon code SUH3RELX   *Normally $149.99 but $19.99 with coupon*

Want to learn a new workout each week?

Join the *Caveman Inner Circle* where a select group of people from across the world complete one of the Cavemantraining workouts together. Not only do you get access to a unique workout each week, you also get access to two kettlebell coaches, and each workout has a progression or alternative, meaning anyone can do them. http://bit.ly/caveman-inner-circle

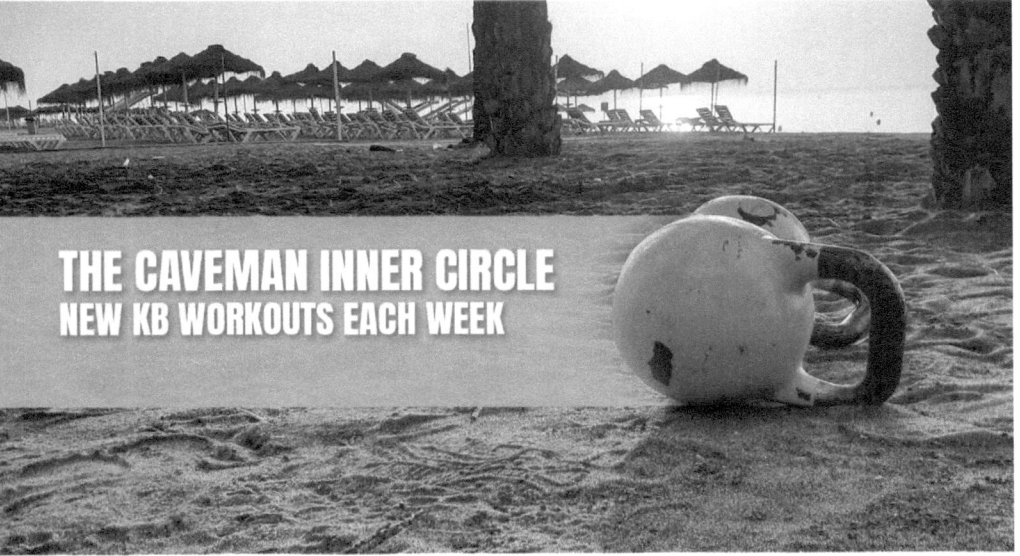

Become a certified kettlebell trainer

Take one of the online Cavemantraining courses and become a certified caveman kettlebell trainer:

- Kettlebell Fundamentals Trainer
- Master The Kettlebell Clean
- Snatch Physics
- CAVEMANROM

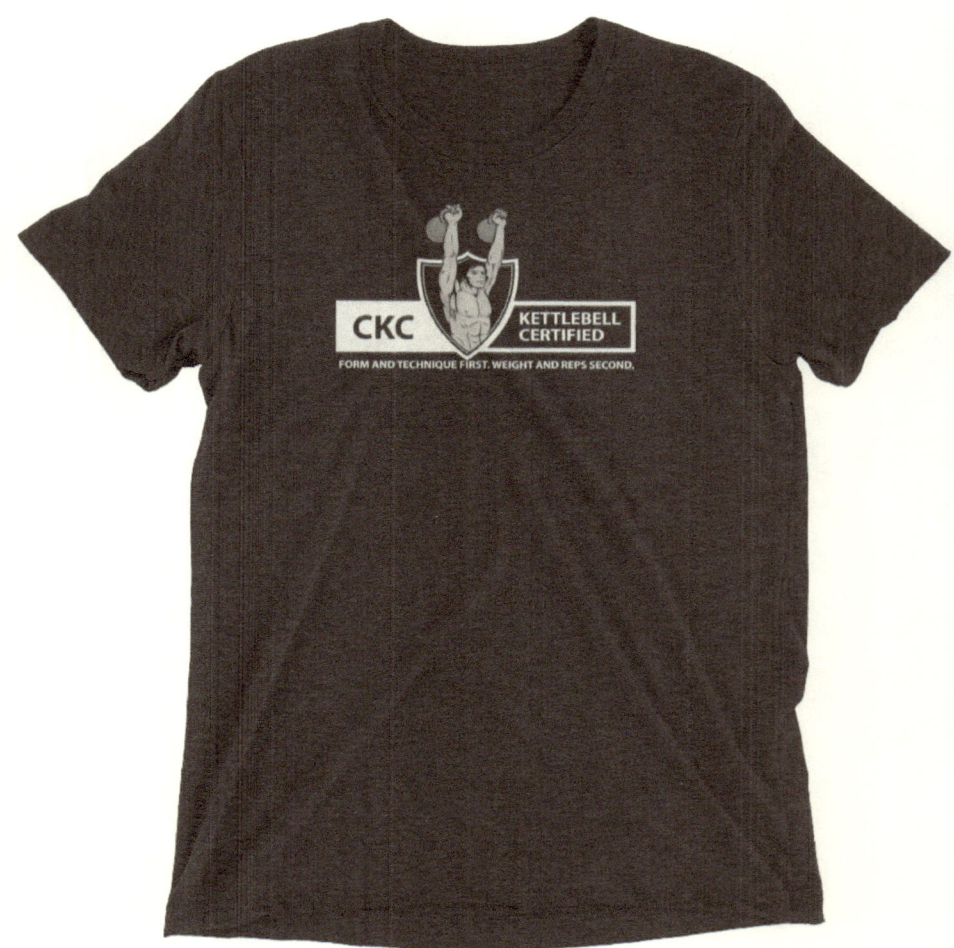

www.cavemantraining.com

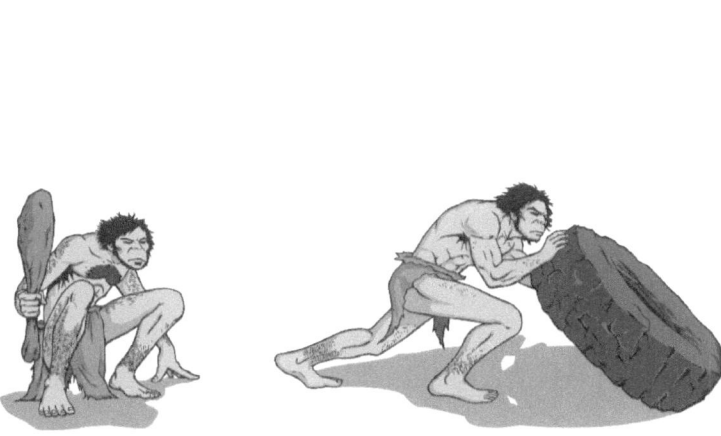
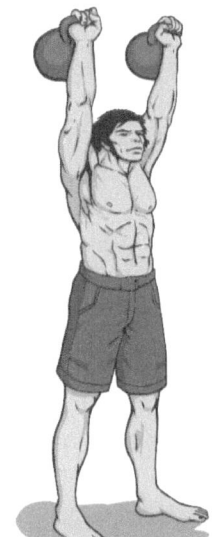